THE POWER OF INTERMITTENT FASTING: UNLOCK YOUR BODY'S TRUE POTENTIAL

Chapters

1. Introduction to Intermittent Fasting
2. Historical Origins and Context of Intermittent Fasting
3. The Science Behind Intermittent Fasting
4. The Benefits of Intermittent Fasting
5. The Risks and Considerations of Intermittent Fasting
6. Popular Methods of Intermittent Fasting
7. Intermittent Fasting and Exercise
8. Navigating Hunger and Cravings
9. Intermittent Fasting for Different Age Groups
10. Intermittent Fasting for Women: Specific Considerations
11. Combining Intermittent Fasting with Various Diets
12. Tips to Make Intermittent Fasting a Lifestyle
13. Intermittent Fasting and its Psychological Effects
14. Frequently Asked Questions about Intermittent Fasting
15. The Future of Intermittent Fasting

INTRO:

Intermittent Fasting is a practice that's been adopted by many health and wellness enthusiasts worldwide. As a health strategy, it has been lauded for its simplicity, adaptability, and effectiveness. The Power of Intermittent Fasting: Unlock Your Body's True Potential is designed to take you on an informative ride through the world of intermittent fasting, focusing not only on the hows and whys of this practice but also on how to adapt it into your lifestyle seamlessly.

This book is not just a compilation of theoretical data and research; it is a practical guide derived from various experiences, incorporating the wisdom of the ancients and the latest scientific findings, and shaped by the struggles and successes of those who have embraced this lifestyle. It aims to give you a comprehensive understanding of intermittent fasting, dispel common misconceptions, and provide you with the tools to successfully implement it in your own life.

But why intermittent fasting? What makes this health strategy stand out amidst the many diets and wellness practices available to us? To answer these questions, the book digs deep into the science behind intermittent fasting, elucidating how it affects the body at a molecular level and why it has such a significant impact on our health and longevity.

But it is not all about science. It is also about history and culture. The practice of intermittent fasting is not a modern trend; it dates back to ancient times and is deeply embedded in various cultural and religious practices. By exploring this historical context, the book provides a rich tapestry that deepens our understanding of the practice and reveals how it has been an integral part of human life for thousands of years.

Interspersed with personal narratives, expert advice, and scientific research, this book presents a balanced view of intermittent fasting, discussing its benefits and potential risks. It does not blindly advocate for this practice; instead, it guides you to make an informed decision based on your individual health and lifestyle needs.

Whether you are a novice to intermittent fasting, someone who has attempted it with mixed results, or a health professional looking for a comprehensive resource, this book is for you. Its evidence-based approach, combined with its practicality, makes it a must-have guide for anyone interested in exploring the world of intermittent fasting.

1. INTRODUCTION TO INTERMITTENT FASTING

Intermittent Fasting (IF) is not a diet in the conventional sense but rather a pattern of eating. It does not specify what foods one should eat, but instead when they should eat them. In this respect, it is more accurately described as an eating pattern.

Most people already "fast" every day while they sleep. Intermittent fasting can be as simple as extending that fast a little longer. It can be done by skipping breakfast, eating your first meal at noon, and your last meal at 8 pm. Then, you're technically fasting for 16 hours every day, and restricting your eating to an 8-hour eating window. This is the most popular form of intermittent fasting, known as the 16/8 method.

Despite what you may think, intermittent fasting is quite easy to do. Many people report feeling better and having more energy during a fast. Hunger is usually not a big issue, although it can be a problem in the beginning while your body gets used to it. No food is allowed during the fasting period, but you can drink water, coffee, tea, and other non-caloric beverages.

Some forms of intermittent fasting allow small amounts of low-calorie foods during the fasting period. Taking supplements is generally allowed while fasting, as long as there are no calories in them.

The basic notion behind IF is simple: by orchestrating your meals to fit within a certain timeframe, you can optimize your body's ability to burn fat, increase metabolic health, and even extend your lifespan. All of these benefits, backed by numerous scientific studies, have led many to adopt this unconventional meal pattern.

The underlying concept of intermittent fasting is nothing new. Humans have fasted for most of our history, whether it's during the typical overnight period, during extended periods of food scarcity, or for religious reasons. What is new is that clinical research on IF's benefits for health and longevity, which has been robust, has been noticed by the public in recent years.

The Power of Intermittent Fasting: Unlock Your Body's True Potential is here to take you through the maze of information surrounding intermittent fasting, providing a clear understanding of what it involves, the different methods, its potential benefits and risks, and how to implement it in your own life. We will explore the science, history, and various facets of intermittent fasting, making it a journey of discovery, self-improvement, and ultimately, healthier living.

In the following chapters, we will delve into the origins of intermittent fasting and its historical significance, the science behind it, and how it impacts your body's physiology. We will examine its potential benefits, from weight loss and improved metabolic health to mental clarity and longevity. We will discuss the popular methods of IF, including the 16/8 method, the 5:2 diet, Eat Stop Eat, and others.

Through this journey, we aim to provide you with a comprehensive guide to intermittent fasting, addressing common questions, clarifying misconceptions, and empowering you with the knowledge to make informed decisions about your dietary habits.

There are different paths within the intermittent fasting journey, and we want to help you find the one that suits you best. So, let's embark on this journey towards a healthier and more vibrant life.

2. HISTORICAL ORIGINS AND CONTEXT OF INTERMITTENT FASTING

Intermittent fasting, while presently a trending health and fitness strategy, is far from a new concept. In fact, it is as old as humanity itself. Our ancestors, the hunter-gatherers, did not have supermarkets, refrigerators, or food available year-round. Sometimes they couldn't find anything to eat, and their bodies evolved to be able to function without food for extended periods.

It's also worth mentioning that our ancestors did not have chronic diseases like obesity, diabetes, and heart disease prevalent in today's societies. Many scientists believe the shift in our eating patterns is a critical factor contributing to these diseases.

Intermittent fasting has also been a part of numerous cultures and religions for centuries. Muslims practice a form of intermittent fasting during Ramadan, a month-long period that requires fasting from dawn until sunset. The Christian practice of Lent also involves a form of fasting, though it's more about eating simpler meals rather than refraining from eating for specific times.

In the Ayurvedic tradition, fasting is often recommended to promote health and balance in the body. The ancient Greeks also recognized the benefits of fasting. Even Hippocrates, the father of modern medicine, wrote, "To eat when you are sick is to feed your illness."

In the Buddhist tradition, adherents were encouraged to avoid eating after noon, effectively resulting in a daily fast. The Jewish practice of Yom Kippur requires a 24-hour fast, and many indigenous cultures have fasting traditions.

It is important to note that these traditional and religious forms of fasting were typically not about weight loss, but about purification and spiritual growth. In fact, the concept of fasting for weight loss is a relatively modern idea.

In the 20th century, fasting began to emerge as a method to treat various diseases, notably epilepsy. This has led to the development of diets such as the ketogenic diet, which is a high-fat, low-carbohydrate diet designed to mimic the metabolic effects of fasting.

Today, as we enter the third decade of the 21st century, intermittent fasting has been rediscovered as a health intervention that can benefit metabolic health, aid in weight loss, and potentially even extend lifespan. It's clear that despite its ancient roots, the benefits of fasting are very much relevant today.

In the next chapters, we will further delve into the science behind intermittent fasting, explore various methods of practicing it, and reveal its potential health benefits and risks. Whether you're interested in the scientific evidence or simply looking for practical guidance, this guide aims to provide a comprehensive understanding of intermittent fasting and its place in a healthy lifestyle.

3. THE SCIENCE BEHIND INTERMITTENT FASTING

Intermittent fasting (IF) has captured the attention of many health enthusiasts not merely because it can aid in weight loss but also due to its multifaceted benefits for metabolic health. The reasons for these benefits are not mystical but deeply rooted in the science of how our bodies function. In this chapter, we delve into the science behind intermittent fasting.

One key mechanism through which IF exerts its effects is by influencing circadian biology, inflammation, and gut health. But, before understanding these complex pathways, let's take a look at the body's physiological response when it experiences a fast.

When we eat, the body spends a few hours processing that food, burning what it can from what you just consumed. This is known as the 'fed' state and is when your insulin levels are high. After this period, your body goes into what is known as the 'post–absorptive' state. Usually, this 'fasted' state begins 8-12 hours after your last meal. It's during this state that the body can burn fat that was inaccessible during the 'fed' state.

As our bodies enter the 'fasted' state, several cellular and molecular changes occur. These include:

1. Insulin levels: Fasting causes the body's level of blood insulin to drop, which facilitates fat burning.

2. Human Growth Hormone (HGH): The blood levels of growth hormone may increase as much as 5-fold during intermittent fasting. Higher levels of this hormone facilitate fat burning and muscle gain and have numerous other benefits.

3. Cellular repair: The body induces important cellular repair processes, such as removing waste material from cells, a function referred to as autophagy.

4. Gene expression: There are beneficial changes in several genes and molecules related to longevity and protection against disease.

When these effects are combined, intermittent fasting results in weight loss, metabolic health improvement, and a range of other health benefits. It's like hitting a 'reset' button on your body that can improve your health and enhance your longevity.

Beyond the metabolic responses, IF can also improve health through other mechanisms. For instance, intermittent fasting can improve your body's resistance to oxidative stress. Additionally, IF can help fight inflammation, a key driver of many common diseases.

Moreover, studies in animals suggest that intermittent fasting can help fight various types of cancer, reduce bad cholesterol, lower blood sugar levels, improve insulin resistance, and even help with brain health.

As we delve deeper into the book, we will explore these benefits in more detail, alongside the potential risks and how to mitigate them. However, it's essential to understand that while IF can be a powerful tool, it isn't a panacea, and individual responses can vary.

◆ ◆ ◆

4. THE DIFFERENT METHODS OF INTERMITTENT FASTING

Now that we've explored the science behind intermittent fasting let's delve into the various methods of implementing it. It's important to remember that intermittent fasting isn't a one-size-fits-all strategy. Instead, there are several different ways to fast intermittently, and the method you choose can depend on your lifestyle, health status, and personal preferences.

1. The 16/8 Method: Also known as Leangains protocol, it involves skipping breakfast and restricting your daily eating period to 8 hours, such as 1–9 p.m. Then you fast for 16 hours in between. This is the most popular method of intermittent fasting, partly because of its flexibility.

2. Eat-Stop-Eat: This involves fasting for 24 hours, once or twice a week. For example, if you finish dinner at 7 p.m. on Monday, you would not eat again until 7 p.m. Tuesday. This method requires a strong will and can be challenging for beginners.

3. The 5:2 Diet: With this method, you consume only 500–600 calories on two non-consecutive days of the week but eat normally the other five days. This form of intermittent fasting has gained popularity due to its relative ease compared to total fasting.

4. Alternate-Day Fasting: As the name suggests, this involves fasting every other day. It may involve not eating at all or consuming a very low-calorie diet (about 500 calories) on fasting days. This method is more extreme and not recommended for beginners.

5. The Warrior Diet: This diet involves eating small amounts of raw fruits and vegetables during the day and one large meal at night, effectively resulting in a form of fasting for 20 hours every day.

Each of these methods can effectively lead to weight loss, as long as you don't compensate by eating much more during the eating periods. Most people find the 16/8 method to be the simplest, most sustainable, and easiest to stick to. It's also the most popular.

It's important to experiment with the various methods and find what works best for you. The best method for you is the one that you can stick to in the long run.

In the following chapters, we will delve deeper into each of these methods, offering insights into their specific benefits and challenges, and provide practical tips to successfully incorporate them into your lifestyle.

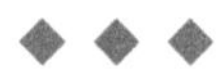

5. THE 16/8 METHOD EXPLAINED

In this chapter, we delve into the most popular form of Intermittent Fasting: The 16/8 method. This method, also known as the Leangains protocol, is favored for its simplicity, effectiveness, and the relative ease with which people can incorporate it into their lifestyle.

The basic concept is to confine your eating period to an 8-hour window, followed by a 16-hour fasting period. A typical schedule might involve finishing your last meal by 8 pm and then not eating again until noon the following day. You essentially skip breakfast and make lunch your first meal of the day.

The reason why this method is called 16/8 is that you are technically fasting for 16 hours each day and limiting your eating to an 8-hour eating window. For most people, this simply means skipping breakfast, and it's a small enough change that people can easily adapt to it.

There are no strict rules about what or when to eat in the 8-hour period, although it is recommended to eat healthy food and maintain a balanced diet. This flexibility is part of what makes the 16/8 method so popular.

Here's a closer look at how it works:

1. Decide Your Eating Window: You need to choose the 8-hour window that works best for you. For most people, this is usually between noon and 8 pm. However, you can adjust the window to fit your schedule. The key is to be consistent with the times.

2. Fast for 16 Hours: During this time, avoid calorie intake. However, non-caloric drinks like water, unsweetened tea or coffee can be consumed.

3. Eat Balanced Meals: During your 8-hour eating window, focus on balanced meals full of vegetables, lean protein, and whole grains. While there aren't specific rules about what to eat, a focus on nutritious food can enhance the health benefits of intermittent fasting.

4. Stay Hydrated: It's essential to stay well-hydrated while fasting. Drinking plenty of water can help manage hunger and keep you feeling good throughout your fast.

5. Listen to Your Body: Pay attention to how your body responds to intermittent fasting. You may need to adjust your plan or eating window to accommodate your body's signals.

It's also worth noting that consistency is key with the 16/8 method, as with any dietary plan. A skipped day or an occasional late dinner won't drastically affect your progress, but consistency is what leads to the long-term health benefits and weight loss that intermittent fasting can provide.

In the next chapter, we will dive into the 5:2 method, another popular form of intermittent fasting that offers a different approach.

6. THE 5:2 METHOD EXPLAINED

In the realm of intermittent fasting, the 5:2 method provides a unique approach to healthy eating. It allows more flexibility than many other fasting techniques, making it a popular choice for many individuals.

The basic concept of the 5:2 method is simple: eat normally for five days of the week and restrict your calorie intake on the remaining two days. The "fasting" days are not days of total fast. Instead, you dramatically reduce your calorie intake for those two days.

On the two fasting days, it is recommended that women consume 500 calories and men consume 600. This equates to approximately 25% of the recommended daily caloric intake. The chosen days should be non-consecutive and spaced evenly throughout the week for optimal results.

Here's a step-by-step guide to implementing the 5:2 method:

1. Choose Your Fasting Days: Pick two non-consecutive days in a week that will be most convenient for you to consume fewer calories. Many people find it easier to fast on weekdays when they are busy with work and other responsibilities.

2. Plan Your Meals: On fasting days, plan meals that are high in protein and fiber as they tend to keep you feeling full longer. A typical meal might include a small portion of lean protein, such as chicken or fish, plenty of green vegetables, and perhaps a small amount of whole grains.

3. Stay Hydrated: Like all forms of fasting, staying well-hydrated is key. Drink plenty of water throughout the day to help manage feelings of hunger and keep your body functioning well.

4. Normal Eating On Non-Fasting Days: On the five non-fasting days, eat balanced meals and snacks as you typically would. There's no need to count calories or restrict certain food groups.

5. Listen To Your Body: Pay attention to how your body feels during this process. If fasting makes you feel weak or dizzy, it's important to adjust your approach. Remember, the goal is to find a sustainable eating pattern that helps you feel your best.

The main advantage of the 5:2 method is its flexibility. Because you are only restricted for two days, it may be easier to maintain than other forms of fasting.

However, it is crucial to approach non-fasting days with a mindset of healthy, balanced eating, not over-indulgence. The goal should not be to compensate for the fasting days but to embrace a sustainable, balanced lifestyle.

In the next chapter, we will explore another form of intermittent fasting known as Eat-Stop-Eat.

7. THE EAT-STOP-EAT METHOD EXPLAINED

The Eat-Stop-Eat method is a slightly more intense form of intermittent fasting and is not recommended for beginners or those with certain health conditions. However, it can be incredibly effective when done properly.

Eat-Stop-Eat involves a 24-hour fast, either once or twice a week. For example, if you finish your last meal at 7 p.m. on Monday, you would not eat again until 7 p.m. on Tuesday. Water, coffee, and other non-caloric beverages are allowed during the fast, but no solid foods.

Here's how you can incorporate the Eat-Stop-Eat method:

1. Choose Your Fasting Day(s): Decide which day(s) of the week will work best for your 24-hour fast. The choice may depend on your schedule, social commitments, and personal preference. Remember, the fast should begin after your last meal of one day and continue until the next day's equivalent meal.

2. Prepare for the Fast: Since this method involves a full day without eating, it's a good idea to prepare yourself mentally. Understand that feelings of hunger will arise but will also pass. Also, consider telling those around you about your fast so they can provide support and understanding.

3. Hydrate and Stay Busy: During your fast, drink plenty of water and keep yourself occupied. Keeping busy can help distract from any hunger pangs.

4. Break the Fast Sensibly: After fasting for 24 hours, be mindful of how you break the fast. Start with a small, nutritious meal, and avoid the temptation to overeat.

5. Listen to Your Body: The Eat-Stop-Eat method can be challenging. Pay attention to your body's response. If you feel overly weak or dizzy, it's important to break your fast and eat something.

It's important to note that while the Eat-Stop-Eat method can lead to significant weight loss, it's not suitable for everyone. This type of fasting can be challenging, especially in the beginning. It is essential to start gradually and consult with a healthcare provider before starting this or any intermittent fasting routine.

In the next chapter, we'll explore the Alternate-Day Fasting method, another approach to intermittent fasting that involves cycling between days of eating and fasting.

8. ALTERNATE-DAY FASTING EXPLAINED

Alternate-day fasting is exactly what it sounds like – alternating between days of normal eating and days of fasting. This style of intermittent fasting is one of the most studied, with research indicating potential benefits for weight loss, longevity, and metabolic health.

However, it is one of the more challenging methods of intermittent fasting and may not be suitable for everyone, especially those new to fasting.

In its strictest form, alternate-day fasting involves a "fast day" where no calories are consumed, followed by a "feed day" where individuals can eat whatever they want. However, many people modify the approach to include about 500 calories on "fasting" days.

Here's a guide to implementing alternate-day fasting:

1. Decide on Your Fasting Schedule: Choose which days will be your fasting days. It can be helpful to create a visual schedule or calendar reminder.

2. Choose Your Caloric Intake for Fasting Days: If consuming no calories on fasting days seems too difficult, you may choose to consume around 500 calories. Consuming these calories as nutrient-dense foods can help keep you feeling fuller.

3. Eat Normally on Non-Fasting Days: On non-fasting days, aim to eat a balanced diet. Although there are no specific dietary restrictions, it's beneficial for overall health to choose whole foods.

4. Stay Hydrated: Hydration is crucial on fasting days. Water, herbal teas, and black coffee (without sweeteners or milk) can be consumed.

5. Listen to Your Body: Alternate-day fasting can be demanding. If you experience dizziness, weakness, or extreme fatigue, it's important to eat something and consult a healthcare provider.

Alternate-day fasting can offer significant health benefits, but it is not for everyone. It requires a level of commitment that some may find challenging. It's essential to consider your lifestyle, your nutritional needs, and your ability to sustain the practice in the long term.

In the next chapter, we'll examine the Warrior Diet, a unique approach to intermittent fasting based on the eating patterns of ancient warriors.

9. THE WARRIOR DIET EXPLAINED

The Warrior Diet is another form of intermittent fasting that has gained popularity in recent years. Based on the eating habits of ancient warriors, who would eat little during the day and then feast at night, this diet proposes a similar cycle of under-eating and over-eating phases within a 24-hour period.

Unlike other forms of intermittent fasting, the Warrior Diet does not completely restrict eating during the fasting phase. Instead, it encourages minimal consumption of small amounts of fruits and vegetables.

Here's a guide to implementing the Warrior Diet:

1. The Under-Eating Phase: This phase lasts for about 20 hours each day, during which you consume minimal amounts of dairy products, hard-boiled eggs, raw fruits, and vegetables.

2. The Over-Eating Phase: This phase lasts for about 4 hours each day, typically in the evening. You're encouraged to eat one large meal at this time. Although there aren't strict guidelines on what to eat, it's recommended to start with vegetables, followed by protein, and finally, carbohydrates if you're still hungry.

3. Hydrate Well: Keeping hydrated is crucial for maintaining energy levels and suppressing hunger. You can drink water, coffee, or tea during the day.

4. Listen to Your Body: The Warrior Diet can be quite extreme due to its long under-eating phase and short over-eating phase. If you feel weak, dizzy, or overly hungry, consider modifying the diet to suit your needs better.

The Warrior Diet encourages a return to "instinctual eating patterns," avoiding the rigidity of calorie counting and meal planning. The main focus is on listening to your body's natural hunger cues and eating in response to them.

In the next chapter, we will look at how to tailor your diet and exercise regimen to complement your chosen intermittent fasting method effectively.

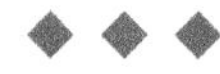

10. TAILORING YOUR DIET AND EXERCISE REGIME

While intermittent fasting is an effective method to control calorie intake and improve metabolic health, it's not a magic bullet. To maximize the benefits of intermittent fasting, it's crucial to also focus on what you eat and how you move.

1. A Balanced Diet: Whether you're eating within a short window, fasting on alternate days, or following the 5:2 method, your diet should be balanced and nutrient-dense. Consuming lean proteins, fruits, vegetables, whole grains, and healthy fats can provide the energy and nutrients your body needs.

2. Exercise and Fasting: Exercise is a critical component of any healthy lifestyle. However, it's important to time your workouts appropriately around your fasting schedule. For instance, some people prefer to exercise at the end of their fast, before their first meal, while others feel better exercising after eating.

3. Hydration: Hydration is key during fasting and exercise. Make sure you are consuming enough fluids, especially around your workout times.

4. Listen to Your Body: Just as with fasting, it's essential to listen to your body when it comes to your diet and exercise. If a particular workout leaves you feeling drained rather than energized, it may not be right for you. Similarly, if you're feeling hungry or unsatisfied after meals, it may be necessary to adjust your diet.

5. Regular Check-ups: Regular check-ups can help ensure that your diet, exercise, and fasting are benefiting your health. Track your energy levels, mood, weight, and other health markers. If you have any concerns, consult a healthcare provider.

Incorporating a balanced diet and regular exercise regime along with an intermittent fasting schedule can amplify the benefits and lead to better overall health. Remember that every person is different, so what works best for others may not work best for you. It's important to find a sustainable and enjoyable routine that suits your lifestyle and health needs.

In the next chapter, we'll discuss the potential risks and side effects of intermittent fasting.

11. POTENTIAL RISKS AND SIDE EFFECTS OF INTERMITTENT FASTING

Intermittent fasting, though beneficial for many, also carries potential risks and side effects. It's important to be aware of these before adopting an intermittent fasting routine.

1. Hunger: Perhaps the most common side effect, hunger can be a significant hurdle during the initial stages of intermittent fasting. Over time, your body will typically adjust to the new eating schedule, and feelings of hunger should decrease.

2. Fatigue and Weakness: Some people may feel tired or weak when first starting intermittent fasting. These symptoms are often temporary and tend to dissipate once your body adjusts to the new eating schedule.

3. Nutrient Deficiencies: If not properly managed, intermittent fasting could lead to nutrient deficiencies. This is particularly true if fasting days involve no food intake or if meals during eating windows lack balance and variety.

4. Overeating: Overeating during eating windows is a common issue, especially when starting out. It's important to remember that intermittent fasting is not an excuse to overeat or indulge in unhealthy foods.

5. Health Risks for Certain Individuals: Certain individuals should approach intermittent fasting with caution or avoid it altogether. This includes individuals with a history of eating disorders, pregnant or breastfeeding women, individuals with diabetes, and those with a history of amenorrhea.

6. Adverse Effects on Social Life: Intermittent fasting can sometimes make social situations involving food tricky. It can be hard to stick to your fasting schedule when meals with friends or family don't align with your eating window.

It's crucial to understand that while many people experience significant health benefits from intermittent fasting, it's not for everyone. Always consult with a healthcare provider before beginning a new dietary regimen like intermittent fasting.

In the next chapter, we'll go over how to get started with intermittent fasting, including setting realistic goals and easing into your chosen method.

12. GETTING STARTED WITH INTERMITTENT FASTING

Starting with intermittent fasting may seem intimidating, but with the right approach, it can be a seamless part of your lifestyle. Here's a step-by-step guide to help you get started:

1. Set Realistic Goals: Before starting, decide what you hope to achieve through intermittent fasting. Whether it's weight loss, better metabolic health, or simply a more structured eating schedule, having a clear goal can help keep you motivated.

2. Choose Your Method: As we've discussed in previous chapters, there are various methods of intermittent fasting. Choose the one that fits best with your lifestyle, daily routine, and health goals.

3. Plan Your Meals: During your eating windows, it's crucial to eat balanced, nutritious meals. Plan your meals to include a variety of foods – proteins, whole grains, fruits, vegetables, and healthy fats.

4. Stay Hydrated: Regardless of the fasting method you choose, staying hydrated is essential. You can drink water, unsweetened tea, or black coffee during your fasting periods.

5. Ease Into It: Start slow. For instance, if you've chosen the

16/8 method, you might start with a 12-hour fast and gradually increase to 16 hours.

6. Listen to Your Body: Pay attention to how your body reacts to fasting. If you feel weak, dizzy, or unwell, it may be a sign that you need to adjust your fasting schedule or eating habits.

7. Regular Check-ups: Especially when starting, it's good to have regular check-ups to ensure your health isn't adversely affected. This is particularly important if you have any pre-existing medical conditions.

Starting with intermittent fasting does not have to be a drastic or challenging change. By following these steps and remaining flexible in your approach, you can successfully integrate intermittent fasting into your lifestyle.

In the next chapter, we will discuss how to stay motivated and handle potential challenges during your intermittent fasting journey.

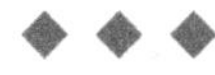

13. STAYING MOTIVATED AND OVERCOMING CHALLENGES

Sticking to an intermittent fasting schedule can be a challenge, especially when starting. Here are some strategies to help maintain motivation and overcome hurdles along the way:

1. Remember Your 'Why': Remind yourself of why you started intermittent fasting. Whether it was for weight loss, improved health, or better meal structure, keeping your goals in mind can help you stay committed.

2. Start Small: If fasting for 16 hours straight feels too hard, try starting with shorter fasts and gradually increase the duration as your body adapts.

3. Plan Your Eating Windows: Planning your meals and eating windows can help you avoid feeling overly hungry and prevent overeating.

4. Stay Hydrated: Staying hydrated can help manage hunger and keep your energy levels up. You can drink water, unsweetened tea, or black coffee during your fasting periods.

5. Incorporate Physical Activity: Regular physical activity can enhance the benefits of intermittent fasting. However, remember to adjust your workout schedule according to your energy levels and eating windows.

6. Get Support: Share your fasting goals with friends, family, or online communities. They can provide encouragement, share their experiences, and even join you in your intermittent fasting journey.

7. Listen to Your Body: If you feel unwell, it's essential to stop fasting and consult a healthcare professional. It's okay to adjust your fasting schedule or try a different method.

Intermittent fasting can become a sustainable part of your lifestyle with patience, planning, and flexibility. It's essential to remember that progress can be slow, and that's okay. The key is to find a method that works for you and stick with it.

In the next chapter, we'll discuss how to maintain an intermittent fasting lifestyle in the long term.

14. SUSTAINING AN INTERMITTENT FASTING LIFESTYLE

Transitioning to an intermittent fasting lifestyle can take time and adjustment, but maintaining it in the long term can offer various health benefits. Here are some tips to make intermittent fasting a sustainable part of your life:

1. Be Flexible: Life is unpredictable, and there will be days where sticking to your fasting schedule might be difficult. It's okay to adjust your schedule as needed. The key is to get back on track as soon as you can.

2. Keep a Food and Mood Journal: Tracking what and when you eat, as well as how you feel physically and emotionally, can provide valuable insights. This can help you adjust your eating windows, meal compositions, and fasting periods to better suit your needs.

3. Stay Social: Don't let your fasting schedule isolate you from social gatherings. If there's a special occasion that doesn't align with your fasting window, it's fine to adjust. Remember, consistency over the long term is what matters, not individual days.

4. Mix Things Up: If your fasting schedule starts to feel monotonous, try a different intermittent fasting method for a while. This can keep things interesting and help you identify the method that suits you best.

5. Get Regular Check-ups: Regular health check-ups are essential, especially when maintaining a specific eating pattern like intermittent fasting. This ensures that your fasting schedule continues to benefit your health.

Maintaining an intermittent fasting lifestyle doesn't mean being perfect all the time. It's about making conscious, health-oriented decisions consistently, while allowing yourself the flexibility to adapt to different situations.

In the final chapter, we will wrap up everything we have learned about intermittent fasting and how to integrate it into your lifestyle for the long term.

15. WRAPPING UP - THE JOURNEY OF INTERMITTENT FASTING

As we close this comprehensive guide on intermittent fasting, let's review and emphasize some crucial points:

1. Intermittent Fasting is not a Diet, but a Lifestyle: Intermittent fasting is not a conventional diet plan but a pattern of eating. It doesn't dictate what to eat but rather when to eat.

2. Flexibility and Adaptability: There are multiple methods of intermittent fasting, all of which can be tailored to suit your lifestyle, preferences, and health goals. This adaptability makes it a sustainable practice for many people.

3. Balance and Nutrition are Key: While intermittent fasting may facilitate calorie restriction, it's not an excuse to consume unhealthy food. It's vital to ensure that your diet remains balanced and nutritious to reap the full benefits of intermittent fasting.

4. Pair with Healthy Habits: Combine intermittent fasting with other healthy habits, such as regular physical activity, adequate sleep, and stress management, to maximize its benefits.

5. Listen to Your Body: Pay attention to how your body responds to fasting. If you feel unwell, consider adjusting your fasting method or consult a healthcare professional.

6. Be Patient: The benefits of intermittent fasting often take time to materialize. Be patient with your body and the process.

7. Get Support: Sharing your journey with others can provide motivation, make the process more enjoyable, and help you stay on track. Consider joining online forums, groups, or having a fasting buddy to share experiences and encourage each other.

Embarking on the journey of intermittent fasting can be a transformative experience for your health and well-being. With the principles and strategies outlined in this guide, you are now well-equipped to navigate the path of intermittent fasting. Remember, the goal is not perfection, but progress and sustainability. Make this journey yours, tailor it to suit your needs, and let the benefits of intermittent fasting unfold.